I0421703

How to Make Hair Grow Faster:

Causes of Hair Loss and Remedies

FAHIM WATSON

DISCLAIMER:

This Book is published in compliance with common decency and for general data reason only. The data contained in this book isn't planned to be prescriptive. Any guidance, dietary recommendations, and a conclusion should go under the course of a certified doctor, beautician or health care proficient.

The data in this Book isn't medicinal counsel and all people ought to counsel their beautician or doctor before attempted any exercises proposed in this book. Any move you make after perusing this data is carefully at your own responsibility.

Table of contents

Introduction:

Since the beginning, hair has assumed a huge job in our general public – it is related to energy and excellence in ladies and virility and manliness in men; so it's nothing unexpected that balding can make numerous people feel reluctant.

Hair has for quite some time been a pointer of both social and expert status and has likewise been worn in various styles to indicate religion. Here are some intriguing certainties about hair since the beginning that you most likely didn't have even inkling.

In Ancient Egypt, the Pharaoh dependably wore a wig to signify his status, while his children wore their hair in buns which were dependable on the correct side of their heads.

Christian clerics and priests once shaved the crowns of their head to symbolize an absence of vanity and their promise of purity

In the book of scriptures, Samson took his solidarity to demolish the Philistines from his long, streaming mane. At

The point when Delilah trims his hair, his quality was no more

Today, hair is as imperative to us as ever, and while numerous individuals are influenced by hair loss eventually in their lives, there are more male pattern baldness medications accessible than any time in recent memory. While many grasp their sparseness, others look for treatment to reestablish their hair to its previous brilliance.

In this book, I will try to present some reason for hair loss and some contrivance to get rid of it.

What is hair loss?

Male pattern baldness is a standout amongst the most troublesome things to adapt to particularly to individuals who are extremely specific about the appearance. However, this doesn't imply that one should surrender his or her life since the individual in question lost the delegated magnificence.

The most exemplary way that individuals can go about male pattern baldness is to realize what causes it. Specialists state that male pattern baldness can either be lasting or transitory relying upon the general status of the individual.

In the language of medical science, Male pattern baldness is the diminishing of hair on the scalp. The restorative term for male pattern baldness is alopecia. Alopecia can be impermanent or lasting. The most widely known type of balding occurs slowly and is recognized as androgenetic alopecia, implying that a blend of hormones (androgens are male hormones) and heredity (hereditary qualities) is expected to build up the condition. Different kinds of male pattern baldness incorporate alopecia areata (patches of hair sparseness that typically develop back), telogen exhaust (fast shedding after labor, fever, or unexpected

Weight reduction); and footing alopecia (diminishing from tight plaits or braids).

Balding ordinarily happens bit by bit with age in both males and female, however, is commonly increasingly articulated in men.

Permanent balding or example male pattern baldness is regular to those individuals whose guardians had something very similar. This is on the grounds that the condition can be innate.

Temporary male pattern baldness then again is normally caused certain ailments and ailments, which debilitates the safe framework and in the end, influences the development of the hair.

About male pattern baldness:

In men, the most widely recognized sort of male pattern baldness is diminishing achieved by "androgens" or "male hormones". Specialists state that men experience design sparseness even at an early age. Also, as they develop more established, balding turns out to be increasingly clearer particularly when diminishing begins at the front and sides of the head.

Numerous men who experience this condition say that the most straightforward, quickest, and least expensive path adapts to male pattern baldness is to overlook it. Since male example hairlessness is unavoidable because of the qualities, it tends to be pointless to stress a lot on something that is inescapable.

This will work for the individuals who have assembled enough certainty not to mind a lot on what other individuals would state about them. In any case, there still the individuals who can't overlook the impacts of male pattern baldness on their lives. For the individuals who are annoyed by balding, the most ideal approach is to make a move, a positive one. Truth be told, you can plan something to fix it through medication and different medicines.

In spite of the fact that these won't thoroughly fix it, these can some way or another moderate the rate of balding. Topical prescription, for example, minoxidil or oral medicine like the finasteride can be utilized. In any case, before you take in any prescription, ensure that you

Counsel your specialist first to keep away from further confusion.

About female pattern baldness:

More than the men, ladies feel more weight when they lose their hair. This is on the grounds that they are increasingly cognizant about what they look like and their certainty significantly relies upon their physical appearance. To stay away from a sentiment of disgrace, there are numerous approaches to adapt to it.

Be that as it may, before doing anything, ensure that you comprehend what the reason for the male pattern baldness is. Visiting the specialist to know the status of the condition and to request accessible treatment alternatives may deal with you.

A standout amongst the most ideal approaches to adapt to male pattern baldness among ladies is to expand the dissemination to the scalp utilizing a delicate and multi-tipped scalp massager consistently. You can likewise utilize milder shampoos or those that are planned to treat diminishing hair and subsiding hairline.

To look increasingly popular, ladies can likewise utilize hair extras, for example, caps to cover uncovered spots or territories that are as of now demonstrating the scalp.

Types of hair loss:

Androgenetic alopecia:

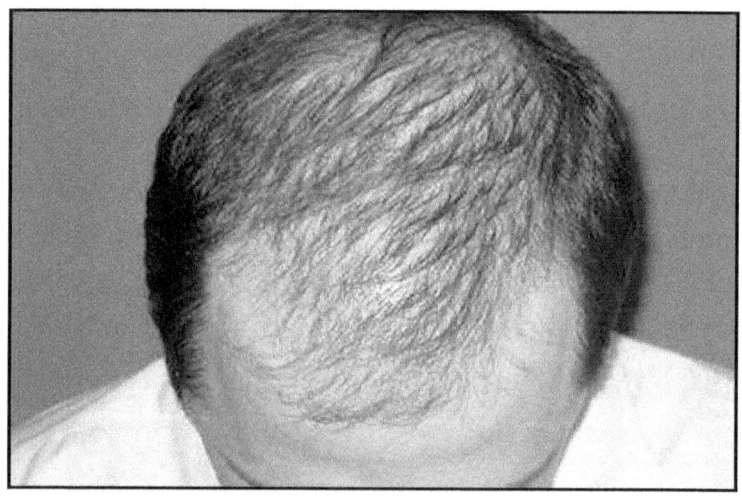

Androgenetic alopecia is the most well-known kind of male pattern baldness, influencing in excess of 50 million men and 30 million ladies in the United States. Regularly known as male example balding or female example male pattern baldness, androgenetic alopecia is genetic

However can be made to do with prescription or medical procedure.

Telogen Effluvium:

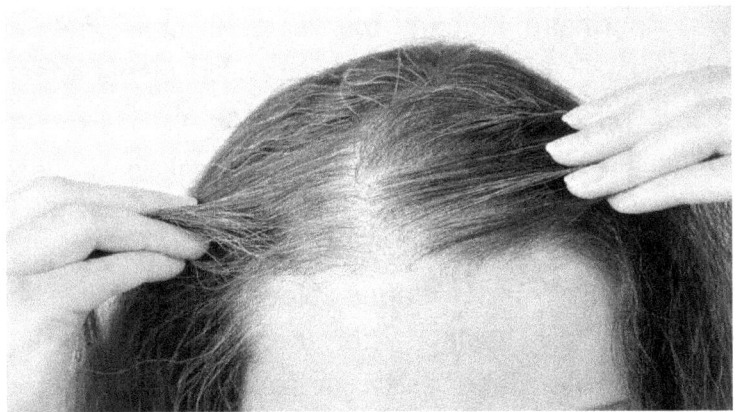

Telogen exhaust, a sort of balding, happens when huge quantities of follicles on the scalp enter the resting period of the hair development cycle, called telogen, however, the following development stage doesn't start. This makes hair drop out everywhere throughout the scalp without new hair development.

Telogen exhaust does not, for the most part, lead to finish hairlessness, in spite of the fact that you may lose 300 to 500 hairs for each day, and hair may seem flimsy, particularly at the crown and sanctuaries.

A medicinal occasion or condition, for example, a thyroid lopsidedness, labor, medical procedure, or a fever, normally triggers this sort of male pattern baldness. Telogen emanation may likewise happen because of a nutrient or mineral lack—iron insufficiency is a typical reason for male pattern baldness in ladies—or the utilization of specific meds, for example, isotretinoin, endorsed for skin inflammation, or warfarin, blood more slender. Beginning or halting oral contraceptives (anti-conception medication pills) may likewise cause this sort of male pattern baldness.

Telogen emanation normally starts three months after a therapeutic occasion. On the off chance that the activating occasion is impermanent—for instance, in the event that you recuperate from an ailment or quit taking the prescription causing the balding—your hair may develop back following a half year. Telogen exhaust is viewed as constant if male pattern baldness keeps going longer than a half year.

For reasons that are hazy to specialists, this sort of male pattern baldness may keep going for a considerable length of time in certain individuals.

Anagen Effluvium:

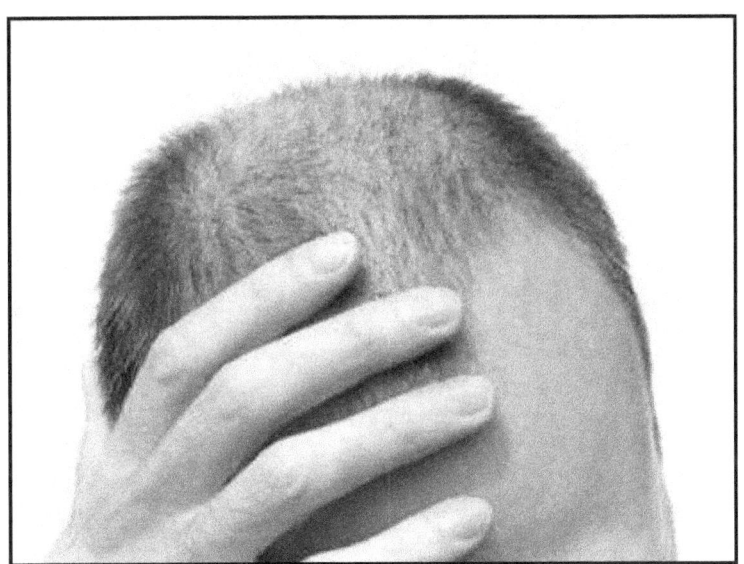

Anagen exhaust is quick balding coming about because of medicinal treatment, for example, chemotherapy. These strong and quick acting prescriptions murder disease cells, however, they may likewise close down hair follicle creation in the scalp and different pieces of the body. After

Chemotherapy closes, hair normally becomes back without anyone else. Dermatologists can offer the drug to enable hair to develop back more rapidly.

Alopecia Areata:

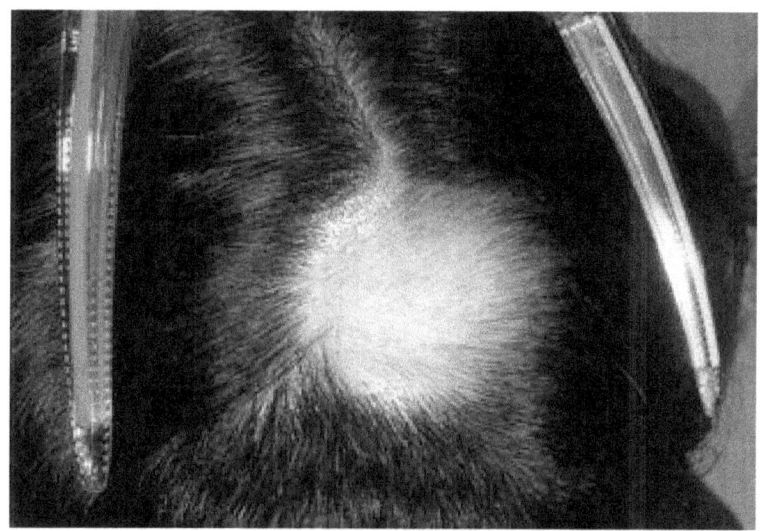

Alopecia areata is an immune system condition, which means the body's safe framework assaults solid tissues, including the hair follicles. This makes hair drop out and keeps new hair from developing.

This condition can influence grown-ups and kids, and male pattern baldness can start all of a sudden and all of a sudden. Hair from the scalp normally drops out in little fixes and isn't difficult. Hair in different pieces of the body, including the eyebrows and eyelashes, may likewise drop out. After some time, this ailment may prompt alopecia total or complete male pattern baldness.

Dermatologists treat alopecia aerate with a drug that may enable hair to regrow. In the event that you are keen on chatting with other individuals who have alopecia areata, NYU Langone has a month to month care group for individuals with this condition.

Tinea Capitis:

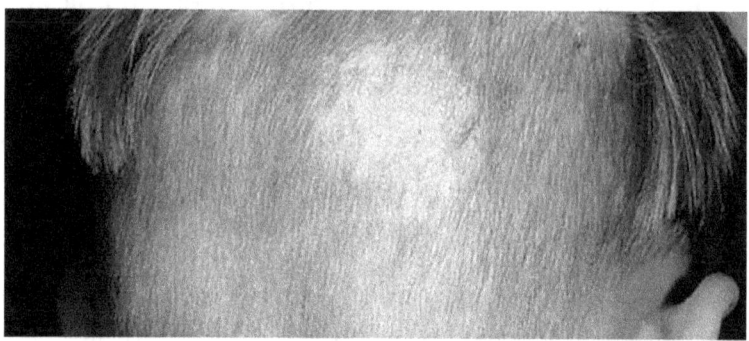

Tinea capitis, additionally called scalp ringworm, is a contagious disease of the scalp that is a typical reason for male pattern baldness in youngsters. This condition makes hair drop out in patches, once in a while roundabout, prompting uncovered spots that may get greater after some time.

The influenced territories regularly look red or textured, and the scalp might be irritated. Bruises or rankles that slime discharge can likewise create on the scalp. A youngster with the condition may have swollen organs in the back of the neck or a poor quality fever because of the invulnerable framework battling the contamination.

Dermatologists can endorse an antifungal medicine taken by mouth to wipe out the growth. In the event that tinea capitis is analyzed and treated early, most youngsters have superb hair regrowth.

Cicatricial Alopecia:

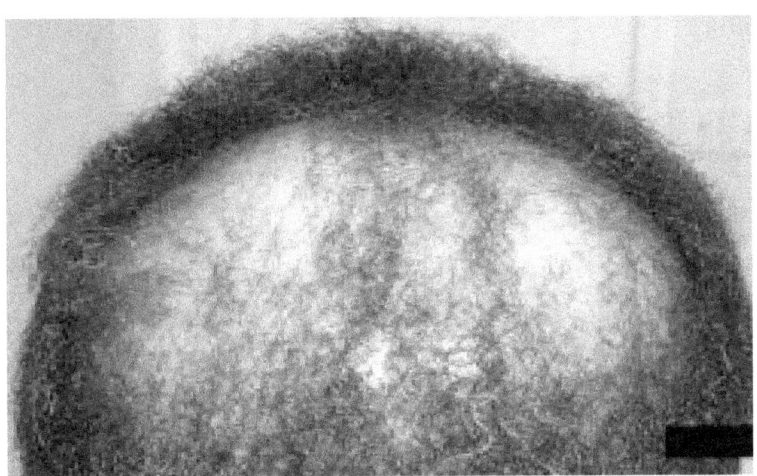

Cicatricial alopecia, otherwise called scarring alopecia, is an uncommon sort of male pattern baldness wherein irritation annihilates hair follicles and causes scar tissue to frame in their place. After scar tissue frames, hair doesn't re grow.

Male pattern baldness may start so gradually those side effects aren't recognizable, or hair may begin to drop out at the same time. Different side effects incorporate extreme tingling, swelling, and red or white injuries on the scalp that may take after a rash. This kind of balding can happen at any age and influences people.

Treatment relies upon the kind of cicatricial alopecia causing your indications.

Lichen Planopilaris:

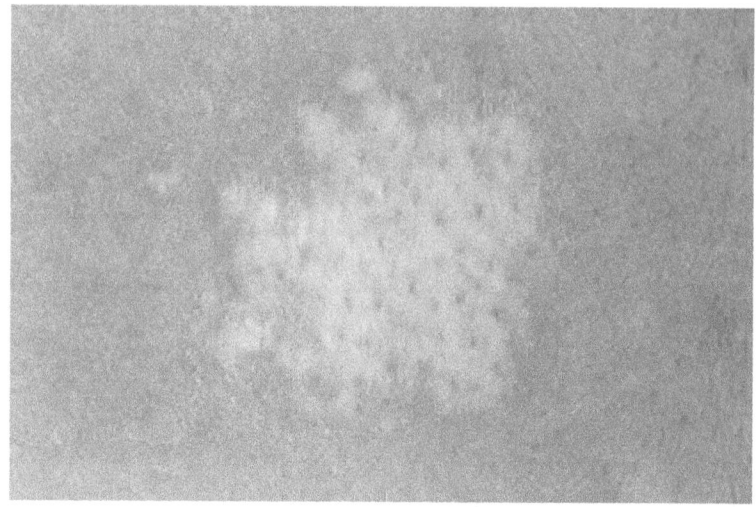

Lichen planopilaris, a sort of alopecia, happens when a typical skin condition, called lichen planus, influences the scalp. Lichen planopilaris may cause a dry, flaky rash to show up on the skin that makes the hair on the scalp drop out in clusters. The scalp may likewise wind up red, chafed, and shrouded in little white or red bothersome, excruciating, or consuming knocks.

Lichen planopilaris isn't normal and influences a larger number of ladies than men. A specialist may recommend the drug to stop the male pattern baldness.

Discoid Lupus Erythematosus:

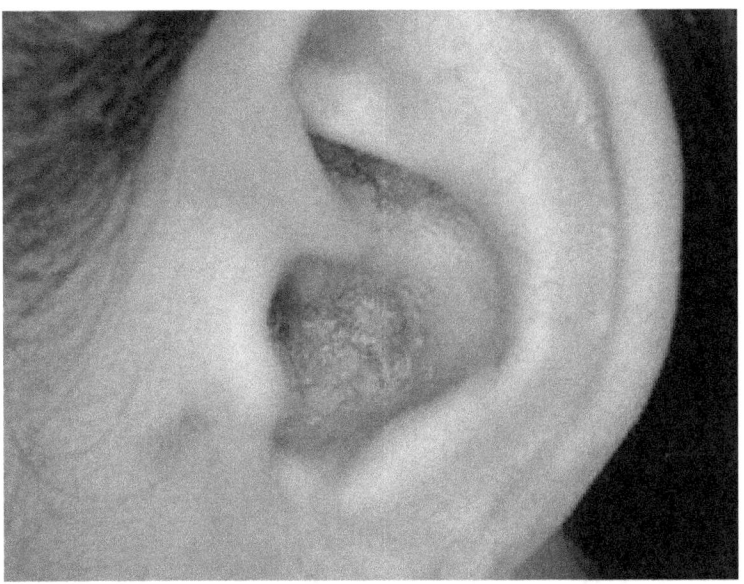

Discoid lupus Erythematosus is a kind of cutaneous lupus, an immune system sickness that influences the skin. It can prompt aroused bruises and scarring on the ears, face, and scalp. Balding is one side effect of the infection. At the point when scar tissue frames on the scalp, hair can never again develop around there.

Folliculitis Decalvans:

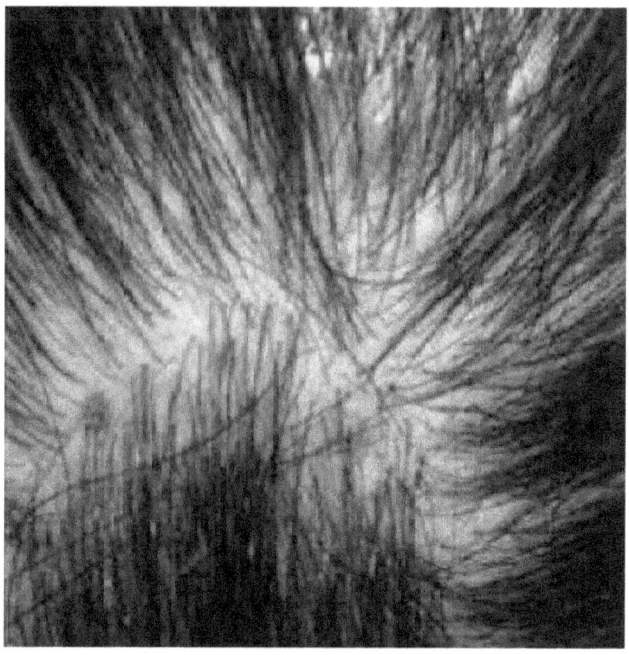

Male pattern baldness brought about by Folliculitis decalvans, an incendiary issue that prompts the decimation of hair follicles, is frequently joined by redness, swelling, and sores on the scalp that might be bothersome or contain discharge, known as pustules. This sort of balding isn't reversible, however, dermatologists can offer medication to control side effects and, on certain occasions, stop the movement of male pattern baldness.

Dismembering Cellulitis of the Scalp:

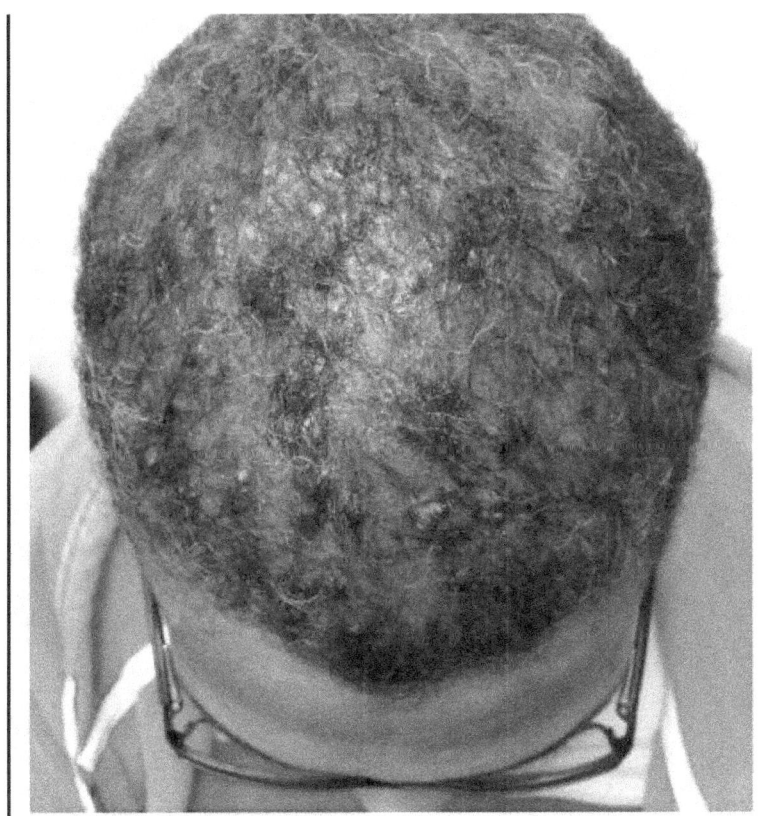

Dismembering cellulitis of the scalp, an uncommon condition makes pustules or bumps structure on the scalp. This condition may likewise cause scar tissue to create, pulverizing hair follicles and causing balding. Drugs may help control indications.

Frontal Fibrosing Alopecia:

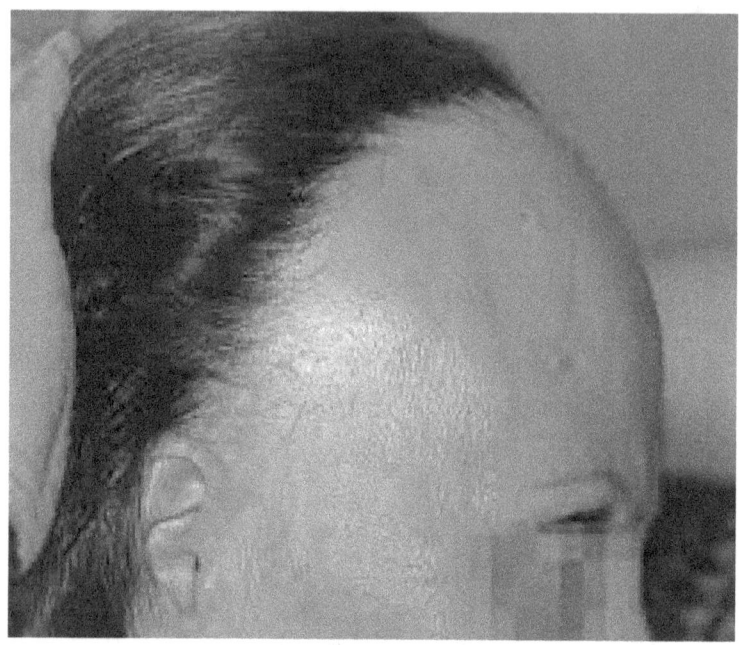

Frontal fibrosing alopecia normally happens in subsiding hairline design and may likewise result in balding in the eyebrows and underarms. Frontal fibrosing alopecia most normally influences postmenopausal ladies. Certain drugs can oversee manifestations and stop the movement of the malady. The reason is obscure.

Focal Centrifugal Cicatricial Alopecia:

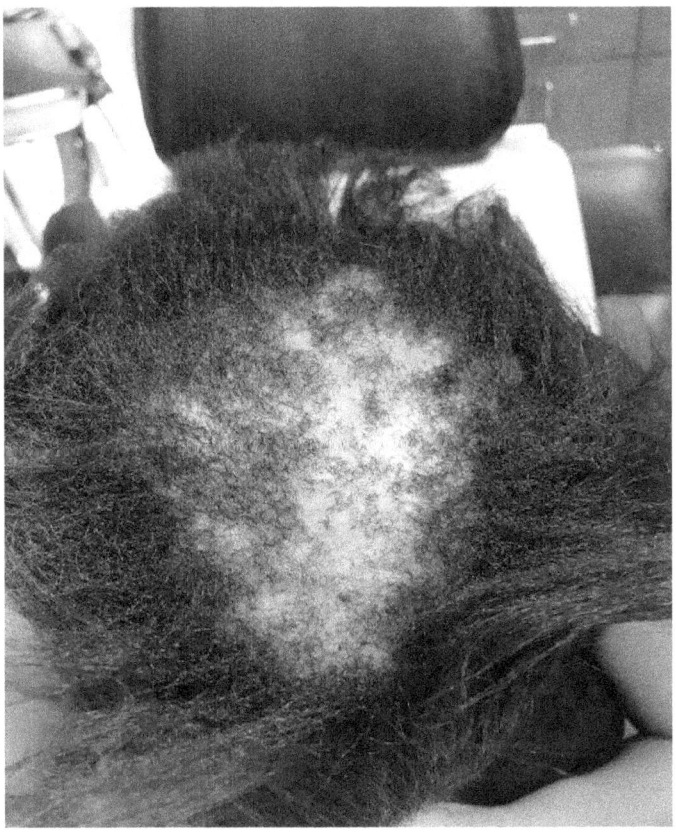

Focal radial cicatricial alopecia may happen because of hair items or styling methods that harm hair follicles. The utilization of hair relaxers, blow dryers, hair curling accessories, and hair augmentations can cause focal outward cicatricial alopecia, as can the way toward making a perpetual wave, or a "perm."

The incessant utilization of oils, gels, or greases can likewise cause this condition, which might be reversible in the event that you quit utilizing these hair items or styling strategies. Our dermatologists may prescribe taking a prescription to enable hair to develop back.

Hair Shaft Abnormalities:

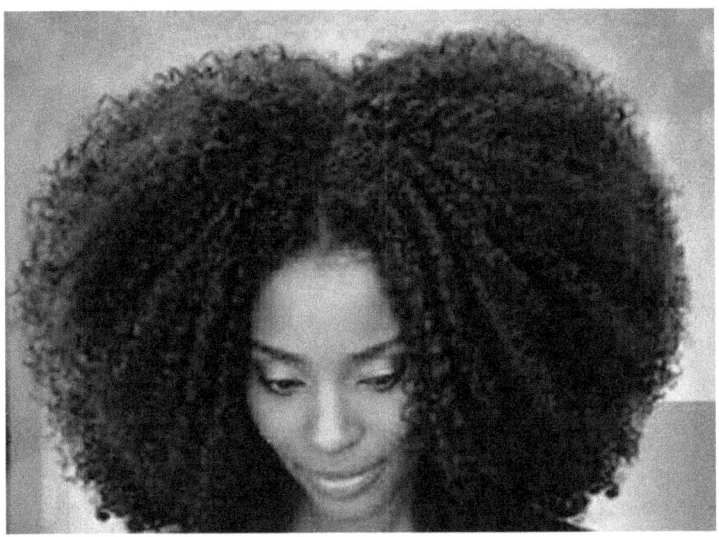

A few sorts of hair shaft variations from the norm can prompt male pattern baldness. These conditions cause strands of hair to thin and debilitate, making them helpless against breaking. The male pattern baldness doesn't happen in the follicle yet because of a break someplace along the hair shaft, which is the noticeable piece of a hair strand. This can result in general diminishing, just as in some little, fragile hairs.

Rolling out basic improvements to the manner in which you style and treat your hair can turn around some hair shaft variations from the norm. Different conditions may require therapeutic mediation. Kinds of hair shaft variations from the norm include:

Free Anagen Syndrome:

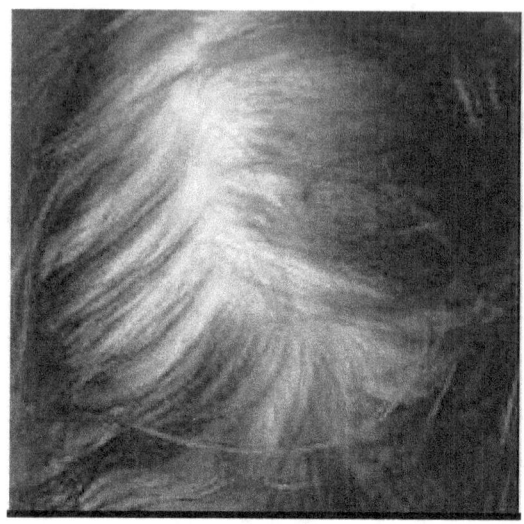

Free anagen disorder, which most normally introduces in youthful youngsters, happens when hair that isn't solidly established in the follicle can be hauled out effectively. More often than not, hair drops out after it has achieved a self-assertive most extreme length. Youngsters with free anagen disorder frequently can't develop hair past a generally short length. The condition all the more usually influences young ladies with light or darker hair.

In individuals who have free anagen disorder, hair can drop out effectively—notwithstanding when it's developing. For instance, male pattern baldness may quicken medium-term in light of the erosion of a pad. The

Reason for free anagen disorder is obscure, however, it might be identified with a turmoil in the hair development cycle that keeps hair from remaining in the follicle.

There are not many dependable medicines, however, the condition will, in general, improve extraordinarily with pubescence, and a few meds may result in more full hair.

Trichotillomania:

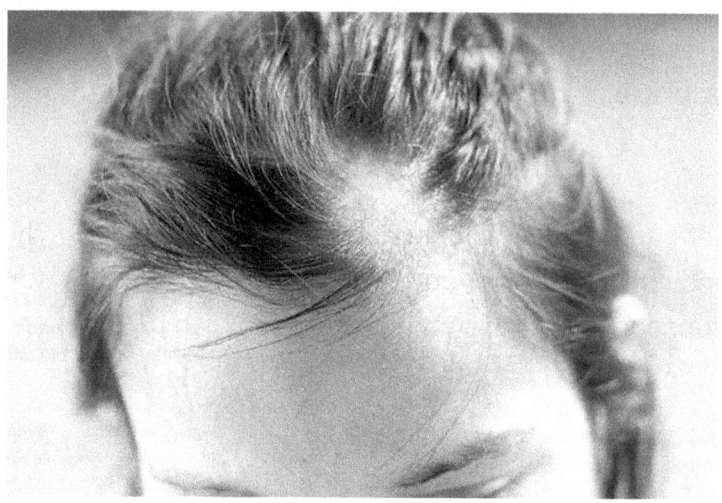

Individuals with trichotillomania haul their hair out and think that it's hard to stop. This outcome in balding on the scalp or somewhere else on the body. Hair regularly returns whether the conduct is ceased, however male pattern baldness can be changeless if the pulling proceeds for a long time.

The best treatment for this condition might be psychotherapy, which may incorporate chatting with an instructor about reasons for pressure and why you want to pull your hair. Our specialists can allude you to a psychotherapist who represents considerable authority in this condition.

Footing Alopecia:

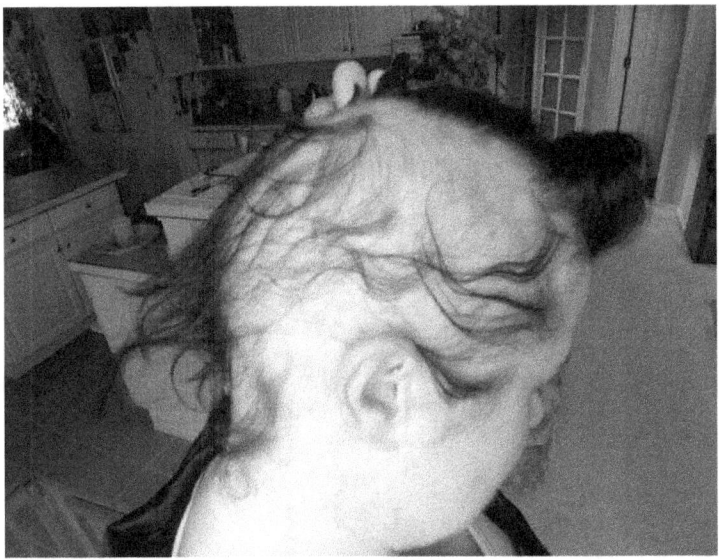

A few hairdos, including tight pigtails and interlaces, pull hair far from the scalp with such power that hair strands are harmed and drop out. Except if the hairdo is changed, footing alopecia may prompt diminishing hair or bare spots. More often than not, hair regrows after you change the hairdo.

Hypotrichosis:

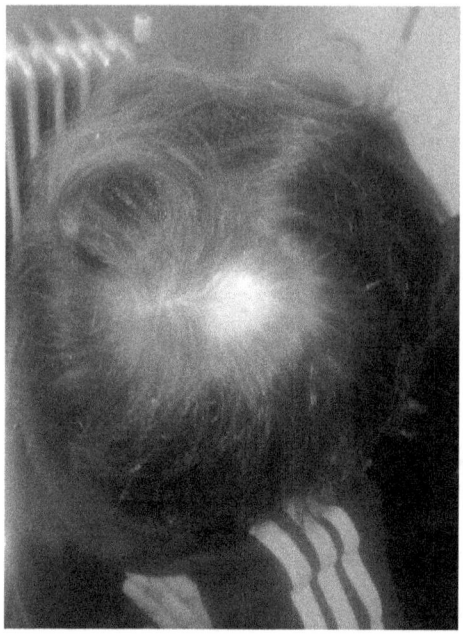

Hypotrichosis is an uncommon hereditary condition wherein next to no hair develops on the scalp and body. Children brought into the world with this condition may have commonplace hair development at first; be that as it may, their hair drops out a couple of months after the fact and is supplanted with inadequate hair.

Numerous individuals with hypotrichosis are bare by age 25. There are not many treatment choices for this condition, yet a few drugs may thicken or regrow hair.

Causes of Hair Loss with their primary solutions:

Reviews state that something that causes individuals to lose their certainty is male pattern baldness. This is on the grounds that numerous individuals can't be certain about the front and even around with others realizing that these individuals are straightforwardly gazing into his or her bare spots.

Specialists state that male pattern baldness or hair loss can be unavoidable to individuals particularly if their families have a background marked by it. These individuals— whose qualities originated from more established ages who are inclined to male pattern baldness—cannot by any stretch of the imagination do much about it since the condition keeps running in their qualities. Be that as it may, for the individuals who don't have it in their qualities and still lose so much hair, right now is an ideal opportunity to stress.

Individuals normally lose around 100 hairs every day. This normally doesn't cause perceptible diminishing of scalp hair in light of the fact that new hair is developing in the meantime. Male pattern baldness happens when this cycle of hair development and shedding is disturbed or when the hair follicle is devastated and supplanted with scar tissue.

Coming up next is a portion of the regular reasons for male pattern baldness. Albeit some of which can act naturally decided, it is in every case best to counsel a specialist since the person can pinpoint what precisely purposes your hair loss.

- ## Family ancestry (heredity):

The most widely recognized reason for male pattern baldness is an inherited condition called male-design hair sparseness or female-design hairlessness. It more often than not happens step by step with maturing and in unsurprising examples — a retreating hairline and bare spots in men and diminishing hair in ladies.

Primary measurement:

Like men, ladies may profit by minoxidil (Rogaine) to help develop hair, or possibly, keep up the hair they have. Rogaine is accessible over-the-counter and is endorsed for ladies with this sort of male pattern baldness.

- ## Physical pressure:

Any sort of physical injury medical procedure, an auto crash, or a serious sickness, even this season's cold virus can cause brief male pattern baldness. This can trigger a kind of male pattern baldness called telogen emanation. Hair has a customized life cycle: a development stage, the resting stage, and the shedding stage. Balding regularly winds up perceptible three-to a half year after the injury.

Primary measurement:

Fortunately, your hair will begin becoming back as your body recoups.

- ## Pregnancy:

Pregnancy is one case of the kind of physical pressure that can cause male pattern baldness (that and hormones). Pregnancy-related male pattern baldness is seen all the more normally after your infant has been conveyed instead of really during pregnancy.

Primary measurement:

If you do encounter male pattern baldness, rest guaranteed that your hair will develop in a few months.

- ## A lot of Vitamin A:

Exaggerating nutrient A-containing enhancements or meds can trigger male pattern baldness, as indicated by the American Academy of Dermatology. The everyday esteem for vitamin A is 5,000 International Units (IU) every day for grown-ups and kids over age 4; enhancements can contain 2,500 to 10,000 IU.

Primary measurement:

This is a reversible reason for male pattern baldness and once the overabundance nutrient is stopped, hair ought to develop regularly.

- ## Absence of protein:

On the off chance that you don't get enough protein in your eating regimen, your body may proportion protein by closing down hair development, as per the American Academy of Dermatology. This can occur around a few months after a drop in protein admission, they state.

Primary measurement:

There are numerous incredible wellsprings of protein, including fish, meat, and eggs.

- ## Male example hair loss:

Around two out of three men experience male pattern baldness by age 60, and more often than not it's because of male example sparseness. This sort of balding brought about by a combo of qualities and male sex hormones, for the most part, pursue a great example wherein the hair subsides at the sanctuaries, leaving an M-molded hairline.

Primary measurement:

There are topical creams like minoxidil and oral meds, for example, finasteride (Propecia) that can end male pattern baldness or even reason some to develop; medical procedure to transplant hair is an alternative.

- ## Female hormones:

Similarly, as pregnancy hormone changes can cause male pattern baldness, so can turning or going off contraception pills. This can likewise cause telogen exhaust, and it might be almost certain on the off chance that you have a family ancestry of male pattern baldness. The adjustment in the hormonal equalization that happens at menopause may likewise have a similar outcome.

Primary measurement:

If another Rx is an issue, switch back or converse with your specialist about other anti-conception medication types. Ceasing oral contraceptives can likewise once in a while cause male pattern baldness, however, this is impermanent. Try not to exacerbate your concern with hair harming magnificence regimens.

• Enthusiastic pressure:

Enthusiastic pressure is less inclined to cause male pattern baldness than physical pressure, yet it can occur, for example, on account of separation, after the demise of a friend or family member, or while thinking about a maturing guardian. All the more frequently, however, passionate pressure won't really encourage the male pattern baldness.

Primary measurement:

As with balding because of physical pressure, this shedding will in the long run decrease. While it's not known whether diminishing pressure can support your hair, it can't hurt either. Find a way to battle pressure and uneasiness, such as getting more exercise, attempting talk treatment, or getting more help in the event that you need it.

• Iron deficiency:

Right around one of every 10 ladies matured 20 through 49 experiences weakness because of an iron lack (the most widely recognized sort of frailty), which is an effectively fixable reason for male pattern baldness. Your specialist should complete a blood test to decide without a doubt in the event that you have this sort of weakness.

Primary measurement:

A straightforward iron enhancement should address the issue. Notwithstanding male pattern baldness, different manifestations of iron deficiency incorporate weariness, cerebral pain, unsteadiness, fair skin, and cold hands and feet.

• Hypothyroidism:

Hypothyroidism is the medicinal term for having an underactive thyroid organ. This little organ situated in your neck produces hormones that are basic to digestion just as development and improvement and when it's not siphoning out enough hormones, it can add to male pattern baldness. Your specialist can do tests to decide the genuine reason

Primary measurement:

Synthetic thyroid prescription will deal with the issue. When your thyroid dimensions come back to typical, so should your hair.

• Nutrient Binadequacy:

Albeit moderately extraordinary in the U.S., low dimensions of nutrient B are another correctible reason for male pattern baldness.

Primary measurement:

Like iron deficiency, basic supplementation should support the issue. So can dietary changes. Discover common nutrient B in fish, meat, dull vegetables, and non-citrus natural products. As continually, eating a reasonable eating routine copious in products of the soil just as lean protein and "great" fats, for example, avocado and nuts will be useful for your hair and your general wellbeing.

- **Immune system related balding:**

This is additionally called alopecia areata and essentially is a consequence of an overactive invulnerable framework. The safe framework considers them to be as remote and targets it accidentally.

Primary measurement:

Steroid infusions are the main line of treatment for alopecia areata, which shows up as male pattern baldness in round patches on the head. Different medications, including Rogaine, may likewise be utilized. The course of the condition can be eccentric, with hair becoming in those days dropping out once more.

- **Abrupt weight reduction:**

Abrupt weight reduction is a type of physical injury that can bring about diminishing hair. This could happen regardless of whether the weight reduction is at the last bravo. It's conceivable that the weight reduction itself is focusing on your body or that not eating right can result in nutrient or mineral lacks. Loss of hair alongside recognizable weight reduction may likewise be an indication of a dietary issue, for example, anorexia or bulimia.

Primary measurement:

Sudden weight reduction appears to stun the framework and you'll have a six-month time of male pattern baldness and after that it redresses itself.

- ## Chemotherapy:

A portion of the medications used to beat back disease, sadly, can likewise make your hair drop out. It obliterates quickly partitioning cells. That implies malignant growth cells, yet additionally quickly separating cells like hair.

Primary measurement:

Once chemotherapy is ceased, your hair will develop back albeit frequently it will return with an alternate surface (maybe wavy when before it was straight) or alternate shading. Analysts are taking a shot at more focused on medications to treat malignant growth, ones that would sidestep this and opposite symptoms.

- ## Polycystic ovary disorder:

Polycystic ovary disorder is an unevenness in male and female sex hormones. An overabundance of androgens can prompt ovarian blisters, weight gain, a higher danger of diabetes, and changes in your menstrual period, barrenness, just as hair diminishing. Since male hormones are overrepresented in PCOS, ladies may likewise encounter more hair on the face and body.

Primary measurement:

PCOS can address the hormone awkwardness and help turn around a portion of these changes. Medicines incorporate eating regimen, exercise, and possibly contraception pills, just as an explicit treatment to address barrenness or diabetes hazard.

- ## Antidepressants, Blood more slender and that's only the tip of the iceberg:

Certain different classes of a drug may likewise advance balding. Increasingly regular among them are sure blood thinners and the pulse medications known as beta-blockers. Different medications that may cause male pattern baldness incorporate methotrexate, lithium, no steroidal mitigating medications including ibuprofen, and conceivably antidepressants.

Primary measurement:

If your specialist establishes that at least one of your drugs is causing male pattern baldness, converse with the person in question about either bringing down the portion or changing to another prescription.

- ## Over styling:

Enthusiastic styling and hair medications throughout the years can make your hair drop out. Instances of extraordinary styling incorporate tight plaits, hair weaves or cornrows just as substance relaxers to rectify your hair, hot-oil medicines or any sort of unforgiving synthetic or high warmth. Since these practices can really influence the hair root, your hair probably won't develop back.

Primary measurement:

Not with standing evading these styles and medications, the American Academy of Dermatology suggests utilizing conditioner after each cleanser, giving your hair a chance to air dry, restricting the measure of time the hair curler interacts with your hair and utilizing heat-driven items close to once every week.

- ## Trichotillomania:

Trichotillomania named a "motivation control issue," makes individuals enthusiastically haul their hair out. Tragically, this steady playing and pulling can really strip your leader of its common security: hair. Trichotillomania regularly starts before the age of 17 and is multiple times as basic in ladies as in men.

Primary measurement:

Some antidepressants might be successful, yet social adjustment treatment is another choice.

- ## Maturing:

It's normal to see male pattern baldness or diminishing of the hair in ladies as they enter their 60s. Specialists aren't sure why this occurs.

Primary measurement:

Experts don't prescribe that this condition be dealt with. That leaves ladies with restorative methodologies, for example, scarves, wigs, and hair styled in order to conceal slim spots.

- **Anabolic steroids:**

On the off chance that you take anabolic steroids—the sort mishandled by certain competitors to beef up muscle—you could lose your hair, as indicated by the American Academy of Dermatology. Anabolic steroids can have a similar effect on the body as polycystic ovary malady (PCOS), as the component is the equivalent.

Primary measurement:

This ought to improve in the wake of going off the medication.

When to seek Medical Advice for Hair Loss:

To certain individuals, they think about their hair as their best resource. In any case, to the individuals who are experiencing balding, this isn't the situation. Rather than being a wellspring of pride and certainty, this very condition fills in as a factor that brings down their fearlessness.

As opposed to basic conviction, age alone does not make the hair fall. Truth be told, an ever increasing number of specialists concur that there are progressively specific factors that reason male pattern baldness both in ladies and men paying little heed to age, race, and status throughout everyday life.

Studies demonstrate that it is sound for individuals to lose in any event 100 strands of their hair consistently. This is on the grounds that this very marvel is an ordinary piece of the hair development cycle. For the most part, the stands of hair the fell are supplanted with another arrangement of hair remains in less the four months or four months.

Be that as it may, individuals who experience more measure of male pattern baldness once a day ought to think about looking for medicinal exhortation. Visiting the specialist about this is significant not exclusively to discover what causes it yet additionally to guarantee that there is no related difficulty alongside the unreasonable male pattern baldness.

Hazard elements of male pattern baldness:

Specialists state that practically all individuals are inclined to losing their hair particularly on the off chance that they don't focus on the hazard variables included. It is said that the essential driver of balding can be followed to heredity.

Individuals whose guardians have sparseness qualities are said to have the most grounded hazard factor. Male pattern baldness for these individuals is very unavoidable since there is no hope with regards to their qualities. The diminishing of hair and retreating hairlines generally show once one age.

Besides heredity, individuals who are experiencing terminal ailments, for example, malignant growth and auto insusceptible ailments, for example, those related to thyroid likewise have more serious dangers for balding on the grounds that the illness themselves debilitate the invulnerable framework and influence hair development.

Taking in prescriptions and medicinal treatment for specific ailments and conditions additionally builds the hazard to male pattern baldness just as alopecia areata, which may cause changeless hair sparseness realized by worry just as different diseases in the earth.

Individuals who don't focus on appropriate nourishment likewise have higher dangers for male pattern baldness particularly the individuals who are low in protein consumption.

Ladies who are pregnant may likewise encounter impermanent male pattern baldness since the nourishment in their bodies is imparted to the developing embryo inside. The individuals who are taking in contraception pills additionally experience this condition on account of the hormonal changes that happen in the body.

Individuals who change hairdos frequently and the individuals who utilize an excess of hair medicines may likewise experience transitory male pattern baldness.

The required therapeutic consideration:

An individual who has in any event three hazard components of male pattern baldness should look for medicinal counsel quickly to avert further confusion. When you go to the specialist, ensure that you call attention to every one of your worries so the individual in question can make the correct analysis and prescribe conceivable treatment choice for you.

The specialist will run a few tests to discover what causes your inordinate male pattern baldness. When every one of the tests has been made, she or he will at that point clarify your condition and will attempt to give you medicine or offer you medications for impermanent male pattern baldness.

Since no treatment can fix perpetual male pattern baldness, for example, those brought about by heredity and ailments, the specialist can give you alternatives to in any event hinder the rate of male pattern baldness.

Diagnosis for Hair Loss:

Prior to making a determination, your specialist will probably give you a physical test and get some information about your medicinal history and family ancestry. The person may likewise perform tests, for example, the accompanying:

Blood test: This may help reveal ailments identified with male pattern baldness.

Draw test: Your specialist tenderly dismantles a few dozen hairs to perceive what number of turns out. This decides the phase of the shedding procedure.

Scalp biopsy: Your specialist scratches tests from the skin or from a couple of hairs culled from the scalp to look at the hair roots. This will help to decide if a disease is causing male pattern baldness or not.

Light microscopy: Your specialist utilizes an uncommon instrument to inspect hairs cut at their bases. Microscopy reveals the potential issue of the hair shaft.

Treatment:

Powerful medicines for certain sorts of balding are accessible. You may probably turn around male pattern baldness, or if nothing else moderate further diminishing. With certain conditions, for example, sketchy balding (alopecia areata), hair may regrow without treatment inside a year.

Medicines for balding incorporate meds, a medical procedure to advance hair development and moderate male pattern baldness.

Prescription:

On the off chance that your balding is brought about by a hidden illness, treatment for that malady will be essential. This may incorporate medications to diminish aggravation and smother your resistant framework, for example, prednisone. On the off chance that a specific prescription is causing the male pattern baldness, your specialist may encourage you to quit utilizing it for in any event three months.

Drugs are accessible to treat design (innate) hair sparseness. Choices include:

Minoxidil (Rogaine):

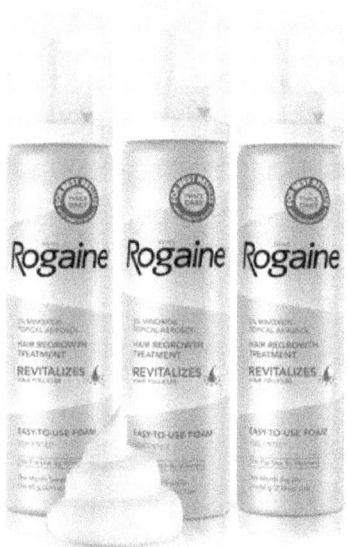

This is an over-the-counter (nonprescription) drug endorsed for people. It comes as a fluid or froth that you rub into your scalp day by day. Wash your hands after application. At first, it might make you shed hair. New growing hair can be thinner and more slender than past hair. In any event, a half year of treatment is required to avert further male pattern baldness and to begin hair regrowth. You have to continue applying the prescription to hold benefits.

Conceivable symptoms incorporate scalp bothering, undesirable hair development on the contiguous skin of the face and hands, and fast pulse (tachycardia).

Finasteride (Propecia):

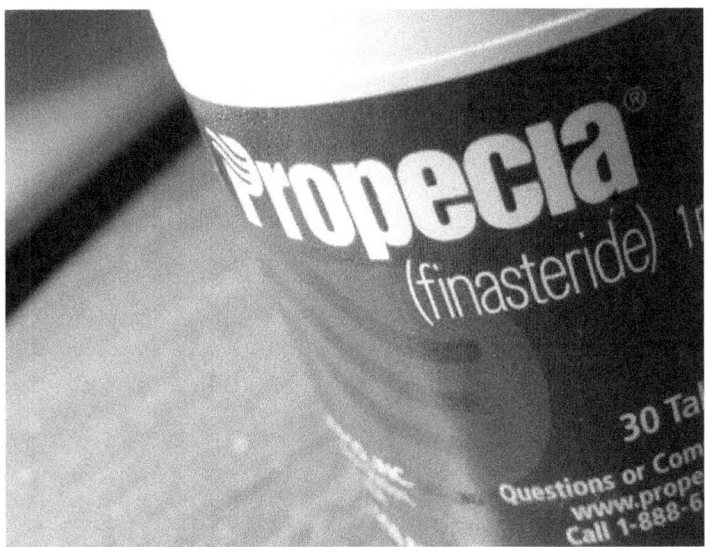

This is a professionally prescribed medication affirmed for men. You accept it day by day as a pill. Numerous men taking finasteride experience a moderating of male pattern baldness, and some may demonstrate some new hair development. You have to continue taking it to hold benefits. Finasteride may not function also for men more than 60.

Uncommon symptoms of finasteride incorporate decreased sex drive and sexual capacity and an expanded danger of prostate disease. Ladies who are or might be pregnant need to abstain from contacting squashed or broken tablets.

Different prescriptions:

For men, oral medicine dutasteride is an alternative. For women, treatment may incorporate oral contraceptives.

Hair transplant medical procedure:

In the most widely recognized sort of changeless balding, just the highest point of the head is influenced. Hair transplant, or reclamation medical procedure, can take advantage of the hair you have left.

During a hair transplant system, a dermatologist or corrective specialist evacuates little fixes of skin, each containing one to a few hairs, from the back or side of your scalp. Some of the time a bigger piece of skin containing different hair groupings is taken. The individual at that point embeds the hair follicle by follicle into the uncovered areas. A few specialists suggest utilizing minoxidil after the transplant, to help limit male pattern baldness. Also, you may require more than one medical procedure to get the impact you need. Genetic male pattern baldness will in the end advance regardless of medical procedure.

Surgeries to treat hair loss are costly and can be difficult. Potential dangers incorporate draining and scarring.

Laser treatment:

The Food and Drug Administration has endorsed a low-level laser gadget as a treatment for innate male pattern baldness in people. A couple of little examinations have demonstrated that it improves hair thickness. More examinations are expected to show long haul impacts.

Clinical preliminaries:

Investigate Mayo Clinic studies testing new medicines, intercessions, and tests as a way to avoid, identify, treat or deal with this sickness.

Planning for your arrangement:

You're probably going to initially carry your worries to the consideration of your family specialist. The person in question may elude you to a specialist who spends significant time in the treatment of skin issues (dermatologist).

What you can do:

Rundown key individual data, including any real anxieties or late life changes. Make a rundown everything being equal, nutrients and enhancements that you're taking. Rundown inquiries to pose to your specialist.

Your time with your specialist is constrained, so setting up a rundown of inquiries will enable you to benefit as much as possible from your time together. Rundown your inquiries from most essential to least significant on the off chance that time runs out. For male pattern baldness, some essential inquiries to pose to your specialist include:

✓ What is likely causing my male pattern baldness?

✓ Are there other potential causes?

✓ What sorts of tests do I need?

✓ Is my balding perpetual or will it develop back? To what extent will it take?

What is the best strategy?

✓ Are there any limitations that I have to pursue?

✓ Would it be advisable for me to see a pro? What will that cost, and will my protection spread seeing an expert?

✓ Is there a conventional option in contrast to the drug you're endorsing me?

- ✓ Do you have any hand outs or another written word that I can bring home with me?

- ✓ What sites do you suggest?

- ✓ What's in store from your specialist

Your specialist is probably going to ask you for various inquiries. Being prepared to answer them may save time to go over any focuses you need to invest more energy in. Your specialist may inquire:

- ✓ When did you initially start encountering male pattern baldness?

- ✓ Has your male pattern baldness been persistent or intermittent?

- ✓ Have you seen poor hair development, hair breakage or hair shedding?

✓ Has your male pattern baldness been inconsistent or by and large?

✓ Have you had a comparative issue previously?

✓ Has anybody in your close family experienced male pattern baldness?

✓ What prescriptions or enhancements do you take routinely?

✓ What, in the event that anything, appears to improve your male pattern baldness?

✓ What, in the event that anything, seems to intensify your balding?

How to prevent Hair Loss:

Sparseness or balding is a standout amongst the most feared circumstances individuals can wind up into. This is on the grounds that this won't just influence their, generally speaking, physical appearance yet can influence their enthusiastic status also.

Specialists classify balding into two sorts—the perpetual male pattern baldness and the transitory male pattern baldness. Lasting male pattern baldness is related to inherited variables. Individuals who have a bloodline that is inclined to hair sparseness can't do much anything about it since it is in their qualities.

The example of hair sparseness or androgenetic alopecia can influence the two people. In men, design sparseness can prompt diminishing hair and retreat of hairlines even at an early age. Inevitably, this condition may lead them to aggregate or fractional hair sparseness.

In ladies, design sparseness may come at a lot later age and does not lead them to add up to hair sparseness. More often than not, the diminishing hair shows at their sanctuaries and hairlines.

With regards to impermanent sparseness, it tends to be brought about by specific factors, for example, sicknesses, taking in prescriptions for specific conditions and experiencing medicinal medications wherein the medication that was utilized takes an excess of a toll on the hair.

There are likewise hormonal changes which can either be brought about by pregnancy or by taking in anti-conception medication pills, hairdos that put an excessive amount of weight on the scalp and prevent it from developing new strands of hair and utilizing hair items and medicines that may disturb the scalp and influence sound hair development.

Avoidance as the key:

Individuals who have dangers for example sparseness can't stop the condition, however, it can slow the rate of balding through different medications. Be that as it may, for the individuals who are experiencing transitory male pattern baldness, counteractive action can be the way to maintain a strategic distance from all-out hair sparseness over the long haul.

Coming up next are a portion of the tips that can help counteract baldness:

Routinely wash your hair with gentle cleanser:

Customary hair washing is a piece of averting male pattern baldness by the method for keeping hair and scalp clean. Doing as such, you are bringing down the danger of diseases and dandruff that may prompt hair breakage or misfortune. Tidy hair also gives the impression to a higher extent.

Nutrient for male pattern baldness:

Nutrients are solid for by and large prosperity as well as useful for your hair. Nutrient A supports the sound creation of sebum in the scalp, nutrient E betters blood course in the scalp to help hair follicles stay gainful and nutrient B enables hair to keep up it's solid shading.

Advance eating routine with protein:

Eating lean meats, fish, soy or different proteins advances hair wellbeing and thus helps control male pattern baldness.

Scalp knead with basic oils:

The individuals who have been encountering balding for a long while must back rub the scalp with fundamental oil for a couple of minutes. It helps your hair follicles stay dynamic. You can incorporate lilac in an almond or sesame oil.

Abstain from brushing wet hair:

At the point when hair is moist, it is in its flaccid state. So refrain from brushing moist hair on the grounds that the odds of male pattern baldness increments. Be that as it may, on the off chance that you should brush wet hair, utilize a wide-toothed brush. Likewise, abstain from brushing hair too much of the time as doing as such can harm hair and increment misfortune. Employ your fingers to harden tangles, not a brush or brush.

Garlic juice, onion squeeze or ginger juice:

Rub one of the juices on your scalp, leave it medium-term and wash it out toward the beginning of the day. Do it normally for a week and you will see the detectable outcome?

Keep yourself hydrated:

The hair shaft involves one-quarter water so drink at any rate four to eight cups of water in multi-day to remain hydrated and for the development of sound hair.

Rub green tea into your hair:

Studies have demonstrated that scouring green tea into hair may help check the male pattern baldness issue. You should simply mix two sacks of green tea in one cup of water, leave to cool and from that point, apply it to your hair. Flush your hair altogether following 60 minutes. To get results, practice this normally for seven days to ten days.

Recognize what is terrible for hair:

In the event that you need to keep hair sound, you should realize how to deal with them. Abstain from scouring your hair dry with a towel. Or maybe, let hair dry normally.

Reduce Alcoholic Beverages:

In the event that you are encountering male pattern baldness than diminish your liquor admission since drinking liquor lessens hair development. So decline or take out liquor to see an expansion in hair development.

Abstain from Smoking:

Smoking cigarettes lessen the measure of blood that streams to the scalp and this causes a decrease in hair development.

Physical movement:

Set aside a few minutes for physical movement consistently. Walk, swim or bicycle for 30 minutes daily helps balance hormonal dimensions, decreasing feelings of anxiety other than lessening hair fall.

De-stress:

Concentrates in the past have discovered therapeutic proof to connection worry with male pattern baldness. De-stress yourself; one of the methods for doing it is by rehearsing reflection. An elective treatment, for example, contemplation and yoga diminish worries as well as reestablishes hormonal parity.

Dodge constant warming and drying:

Try not to expose your hair to visit, consistent warming and drying techniques. Warmth debilitates hair proteins, and steady warming and drying can prompt shortcoming and delicacy that causes male pattern baldness.

Keep your head sweat free:

Men with slick hair, experience dandruff during summer because of perspiring and the odds of hair fall increments. Utilizing shampoos that contains aloe vera and neem can keep the head cool and keep from dandruff

Additionally, men who wear cap experience significant balding in summer. As the perspiration gathers in the pores and debilitates hair roots causing balding in men. So wearing a scarf/bandanna over your hair or a terry material headband can forestall male pattern baldness.

Change your hairstyle (for men with long hair):

On the off chance that you are losing your hair recently, you should extricate up your hair. Hairdos, for example, pigtails, twists and counterfeit haircuts pull hair or pull hair follicles, and can in the long run reason hairlessness.

Deal with your wellbeing:

Medical issues are harbingers of male pattern baldness. Guarantee you manage constant diseases, high fevers, and contaminations appropriately to guarantee sound hair.

Keeps a watch taking drugs:

Certain prescriptions may have reactions, one of which could be male pattern baldness. Counsel a specialist to get some information about the conditions that you may have. Fill him in as to whether the medicine is causing balding and if that is the situation, request that he change the drug.

Avoid synthetics:

Brutal synthetics and lasting hair shading items could be harming hair wellbeing. When you are encountering male pattern baldness, it is exhorted not to shading your hair.

Timetable meetings with specialists normally:

There are numerous wellbeing conditions, especially skin-related conditions, that cause changes in hormonal adjust which thus lead to male pattern baldness. Ensure you see a specialist normally for your basic diseases and conditions.

Home Remedies for Hair Loss:

It is basic for individuals to lose strands of their hair particularly when it is wet or when they brush it all the time. Specialists state that there is a requirement for certain strands of hair to fall so these can be supplanted with another arrangement of hair strands.

The normal strands ought to, at any rate, be a hundred. Once there is abundance in this gauge, at that point, you may experience the ill effects of male pattern baldness.

In the event that you think you are experiencing male pattern baldness, the most ideal approach to manage it is to visit a specialist to guarantee that the person will give appropriate determination. Individuals who are inclined to perpetual hair loss brought about by qualities or those that are brought about by skin issue, they ought to counsel a specialist what treatment alternatives are accessible.

Be that as it may, for the individuals who are encountering brief male pattern baldness, they can manage it regardless of whether they are at home. The accompanying home cures can be utilized to manage male pattern baldness at home:

The marvels of the back rub:

Antiquated individuals have demonstrated that back rub can help stop unnecessary hair fall since it makes the follicles of the hair more grounded. Besides that, it is additionally great since it helps hair development by putting the appropriate measure of weight on the scalp.

More often than not, this is done physically. You can do it without anyone else's help or you can request that someone rub your scalp at home. On the off chance that you don't have enough vitality to do a manual back rub without anyone else scalp, you can pick electric hair to knead accessible in many health stores.

Hot oil medicines:

Specialists state that individuals who are inclined to balding can profit such a great amount from hot oil medicines in light of the fact that these can help avert falling hair and can fix minor scalp issues too. To get viable outcomes, in any event, three medications are exhorted week by week.

You can do this at home with the utilization of a shower top. You can purchase prepared to use hot oil medications that contain oils of a few herbs, for example, sesame, olive, and coconut. For all the more loosening up hot oil treatment at home, settle on those that contain fundamental oils, for example, thyme, lavender, and others.

Aloe vera extricates:

Considered as a "wonder plant", aloe vera is mainstream to numerous individuals—particularly those living in tropical nations—as a solution for balding.

Contingent upon the degree, aloe vera can be utilized as a cleanser by utilizing a new mash that is legitimately connected on the hair and scalp, as a hair tonic alongside different herbs, and a beverage or oral aloe juice for the body to retain its fixings quicker.

Blend of cinnamon and nectar:

Numerous individuals state that one of the viable home solutions for male pattern baldness is the blend of cinnamon powder and nectar with olive oil in light of the fact that these contain properties that make the scalp just as the hair more grounded.

By thinking of glue that can be connected straightforwardly to from the hair's underlying foundations down to the scalp, individuals can utilize it before they utilize their preferred cleanser.

Concentrates of ginger:

A bit of ginger, when cleaved and legitimately connected to the zone of the head that has uncovered spots, can be a viable hair solution for male pattern baldness since it helps the solid development of hair follicles. Since it very well may be rotten, you can likewise utilize its concentrate that is joined with a fine lead powder to get the best outcomes.

Natural Home Conditioner:

To keep up sparkly bolts and to expel any buildup, pursue this hair upkeep formula. Don't neglect to attempt a fix test first to guarantee you have no hypersensitive responses.

Wash hair with an explaining cleanser. After cleanser is flushed and is crushed to evacuate however much water as could reasonably be expected, drench your hair in a weakened blend of water and apple juice vinegar (ACV). Utilize 2 cups of water with 2 tablespoons of apple juice vinegar. Pour the blend of ACV and water on the scalp from the roots at that point down to the tips of the hair or on the other hand, utilize a splash bottle. Leave weakened blend on the hair for around 5-10 minutes. Spread your wavy signs with a plastic top and wrap the head with a warm towel. Flush hair with warm water altogether to guarantee all or any development has been expelled from the hair. This hair treatment should be possible like clockwork or perhaps once per month - relying upon the state of the hair. This helpful formula adds sheen and delicateness to your hair. Utilized as a hair flush, vinegar kills the antacid left by shampoos. This formula can be utilized for all hair types to add sheen and non- abrasiveness to your hair. Ensure you get enough protein in your eating routine. Dairy items and red meat are fundamental to having fun wavy hair. An absence of protein in your eating regimen will influence the shade of your hair. For model, in the event that you do need protein, your hair shading will change in shading from dark to orangey red.

Steam Treat Your Hair:

Steam medications advance the simple retention of water and lotions from conditioners to profoundly enter the hair shaft. Utilize a steam treatment particularly when profound molding your hair.

Just utilize a warm towel to cover wet hair after a cleanser wash or a steam top for 20-30 minutes. Tail it with a warm than a cool flush. The glow of the steam will open up the pores and help evacuate any soil on the hair and scalp. The cool wash will close the pores and hair shaft to further shield the hair from any harm. This is a fantastic everyday practice to do each two weeks.

Lift your Self-Confidence in spite of Hair Loss:

Numerous individuals are certain about dealing with themselves before other individuals since they are happy with the manner in which they look. Yet, for individuals who are encountering male pattern baldness, being sure about the front of others can be a troublesome thing.

This is on the grounds that they can't resist the opportunity to believe that the general population they are managing just spotlight on their falling crown of greatness and not on what they are stating.

While the facts demonstrate that male pattern baldness can incredibly influence one's by and large physical appearance, this isn't sufficient motivation to lose self-assurance completely. In the event that you are one of those people who are gradually losing their self-assurance because of male pattern baldness, a standout amongst the best things that should be possible is figuring out how to adapt to it.

Adapting to male pattern baldness can begin with the acknowledgment that you may truly be experiencing a condition that is truly out of your control.

Specialists state that hairlessness or male pattern baldness can be ordered into two—lasting male pattern baldness and impermanent male pattern baldness. Individuals who are experiencing perpetual male pattern baldness are the individuals who have the condition in their qualities.

Since it is genetic, one can't generally do as much about it yet to figure out how to acknowledge it and attempt to look for elective cures that can slow the pace of losing hair.

Another condition where one can't generally take care of balding is in the event that they are experiencing immune system diseases, for example, malignant growth, thyroid entanglements or lupus. Individuals who need to experience medicines are additionally in more serious danger of losing hair quick.

Individuals who are enduring impermanent male pattern baldness are the individuals who experience hormonal changes, for example, pregnancy in ladies or taking in conception prevention pills just as the individuals who put an excessive amount of weight on their scalp by changing hairdos regularly or those that are utilizing hair items that are destructive to the hair.

Knowing the reason for your male pattern baldness can enable you to adapt to it simpler. Obviously, you can't decide this all alone so you need to visit your specialist to address your worry. When the person had the last analysis, you would now be able to request accessible treatment or alternatives that will work for you.

Tips to be increasingly sure

Here are some sound bites ensured to add length to your twists. (In any case, you need to eat them all the time).

- Almonds
- Raisons
- Oranges
- Entire grain SnackBar
- Strawberries

- Fish liver oils
- Liver
- Dim green vegetables
- Yellow Vegetables
- Pumpkin
- Dairy Products
- Prunes
- Chicken
- Hamburger Salmon
- Ocean growth
- Citrus Fruits like oranges and grapefruits
- Blueberries
- Sardines and Salmon
- Lentils
- Eggs
- Wheat grain and Wheat germ
- Watercress, Spinach, Kale
- Darker Rice
- Melon

ONE LAST TIP FOR YOU

What Ingredients to Avoid In Shampoos:

Everybody adores having flawless haircuts that copy an expert looks that you have when you leave the salon. The principal issue is that numerous individuals end up with dry and harmed hair before they know it and your cleanser could be the principal offender. There are wide assortments of fixings that are incorporated into conventional cleanser equations that have been broadly contemplated and have appeared be harming to the hair and skin of individuals that utilization them.

The following is an instructive manual to show you the various fixings that you ought to stay away from in your shampoos and the fixings that you ought to search for.

Fixings to Avoid:

On the off chance that you've done any examination into synthetics and aggravates that are awful for your hair, you've without a doubt known about the 3 hair executioners:

• Sulfates

• Parabens

• Phthalates

• **Sulfates:**

Ordinarily known as the fixings that are in charge of making the thick bubbly foam in shampoos, sulfates were initially intended for modern chemicals. These synthetic compounds are in charge of slicing through oil and grime in request to dispose of the majority of the oil in your hair. The fundamental issue is that your hair needn't bother with the majority of its oil evacuated, just the abundance that is made for the duration of the day. The more oil that is expelled from your hair, the more oil your body is going to deliver to compensate for what it doesn't have which results in heavier and greasier strands than at any other time. There are additionally hurtful results that have been found within sulfates, counting 1, 4-dioxane, which has been connected to kidney and liver harm.

- **Parabens:**

Parabens are commonly known to be antifungal and antibacterial specialists that help to clean various surfaces, yet in an inconceivably undesirable manner. Various examinations have demonstrated that parabens have been found within tumors and can be identified with noteworthy changes in hormone capacities, especially in more youthful young ladies. One of the biggest worries that buyers have with parabens is that they are found in pretty much every kind of kids' cleanser since they are such solid additives that keep equations better for more. There has been some theory around whether formaldehyde is one of the fundamental gases that are radiated from parabens after they have been put away for a brief timeframe.

- **Phthalates:**

Phthalates are regularly found within plastics however they can likewise be utilized to make most of the scents that you have in your shampoos. These fixings are on an assortment of records in various nations that point legitimately to cancer-causing agents, the things that are in charge of making malignancy, what's more, different infirmities. Different investigations have noted phthalates are in charge of disturbing the endocrine capacities in young ladies and intensifying the side effects of asthma in the two kids and grown-ups. Truth be told, California prohibited the utilization of phthalates in kids' toys dating back to 2009. The principle approach to ensure that you don't succumb to these destructive segments is to peruse the fixings list on your cleanser.

With regards to a sulfate free cleanser item, here is the thing that you have to know:

- ✓ A sulfate-free cleanser is a cleanser that does not contain sodium lauryl sulfate (SLS). SLS is otherwise called sodium lauryl sulfate

- ✓ In the event that you check the fixings posting for some business cleaning also, cleanliness items, you will find that SLS is every now and again recorded as a fixing.

- ✓ SLS is intended to help evacuate sleek buildups, among other things.

- ✓ Despite the fact that the sulfate part to these cleanliness items does not have cancer-causing properties, the synthetics do can possibly cause various issues.

✓ A portion of the potential issues related to SLS incorporates bothering to the scalp, the likelihood of fundamental oils being stripped, and the hair winding up excessively dry.

✓ Individuals respond to sulfates in an unexpected way. Some are very hypersensitive, while others just experience a portion of the issues referenced above to a gentle degree. Some don't encounter any of the issues referenced above to any huge degree at all.

✓ For the individuals who have delicate skin or solid sulfate sensitivities, a sulfate free cleanser could demonstrate to be actually what they've been looking for in a cleanser item.

Conclusion:

I have composed this book with a great deal of commitment and meeting of some known individual. I figure this book will doubtlessly help those individuals who are experiencing sparseness and furthermore losing their hair to a degree sum. It very well may be an incredible purchase for you and a gift for your dearest one. On the off chance that you like this book, give your profitable audits to promote improvement.